Don't L
Your Wig...

AND OTHER THINGS THE ONCOLOGIST
NEVER TOLD YOU!

Don't Let the Cat Get Your Wig…

AND OTHER THINGS THE ONCOLOGIST NEVER TOLD YOU!

BY
LAUREN BROWER

Illustrations by
Brandi Gordon

eBookstand Books
http://www.ebookstand.com

Published by
eBookstand Books
Division of The Magnum Group
Auburn, Ca 95604

ISBN 1-58909-078-0

Printed in the United States of America

Table of Contents

Introduction

Chapter One: Surgery and Diagnosis   3

Chapter Two: Chemotherapy   15

Chapter Three: Radiation   27

Chapter Four: Chemo the Sequel   35

Chapter Five: Random Moments of Joy   43

Introduction

From the very moment I was diagnosed with Breast Cancer at age 34, I felt a drive, almost compulsion, to write about my experiences. I felt that in some way I had a responsibility to prepare others who might follow in my footsteps or that may have a family member struggling with this disease. So I set out to lay the framework for this "book".

I read and researched many books on the subject and realized that there is a great deal of material out there on coping with the disease and managing the side effects. I began to worry that there was no approach that I could take that would provide a fresh perspective. What could I say that hadn't been said before? Then through a series of events I began to realize the element that I might be able to provide was humor.

Laugh? At such a serious disease? Surely I must not understand the severity of the illness! On the contrary, I understand quite well. I understand the fear of losing one's life at a young age and dealing with the fear of the unknown. I watched my mother struggle with the same disease and fears as well. It came to me most distinctly through a phone call from a friend, that using humor to share some valuable lessons about coping could be exactly what many of us need. Maybe it can teach us the most valuable lesson of all, to laugh at ourselves, to laugh at adversity. Perhaps then we can become the self-actualized, healthy people we deserve to be.

I feel it prudent to add that I have the fondest memory of a fellow high school chum who was the proud bearer of an "artificial foot". For someone of high school age such an encumbrance could be laughable to his peers, but he used it to his advantage. Having the gift of a theatrical personality, he would hide it in lockers and make allusions to having his "foot in his mouth". There were numerous games to be played. Not one of us laughed at him, we did find however that he made us laugh. Additionally, NONE of us were uncomfortable with his physical challenge, which really made him less challenged and more special. So perhaps the humor here can also serve a similar purpose. Perhaps it can make a difficult subject more approachable, so that we can face our fears.

I also want to state that it isn't my intention to write "knock your socks off" comedy here. Rather, I have tried to find humor in challenging situations. You will find a few humorous anecdotes in this book and you might find some real advice and help in preparing for your own struggle. If you do, then I have accomplished my goal. There is one additional point I feel it necessary to make. The suggestion that we find humor in these events that happen to us, is merely that. Its just a suggestion. It is also quite normal and necessary to cry. I don't pretend that this struggle is easy and I don't wish to make light of a serious illness. I've written this book in the voice of a survivor speaking to the newly diagnosed. It is only my desire to make their struggle easier with a little laughter. All I suggest is that each and every one of you take good care of yourselves and your loved ones in whatever way is comfortable and healthy for YOU.

Chapter One: Surgery/Diagnosis

Has everyone seen my boob?!

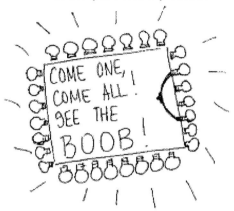

There is a phenomenon that occurs during diagnosis and in the weeks that follow, when suddenly that which is extremely personal seems to become everyone's business. Just because of the nature of the illness your breast seems to become community property. There were family members who wanted to "see", doctors who needed to "see", and people who may not have desired to "see" but got flashed anyway because I suddenly became used to baring my chest to the viewing public. Alright, it wasn't like I was dancing topless, but I certainly had to get used to the idea that my breast was now a subject of interest for a legitimate reason. The sooner I was able to accept this as either concern or professional necessity rather than an invasion of privacy the easier it was for me to cope with the situation.

Being comfortable with your body and having a sense of humor will serve you well. It may seem too soon after the shock of being diagnosed for some to be able to laugh, but the sooner a person can do so, the faster they will be on the road to recovery. My sense of humor almost took over without my awareness at times and it probably shocked people. One day early in my diagnosis I found myself chiding my radiation oncologist, who commented that my left breast was the "affected" one while the right breast was "unremarkable". "Says who?" I asked with wry smile. Since then we have had a fabulous rapport. The doctors seem to appreciate a sense of humor in their patients. They see the healthy attitude and know that they have someone who will work with them.

4

I do have to mention that my surgeon did such a fabulous job that I am still apt to show any curious parties his exceptional work. This is after all, the man who is rumored to have done a biopsy on a pool table. You can't get any cooler than that. He is still amazed at his own genius every time I go back for a follow up. He's entitled to gloat.

Hey, has everyone seen my boob?!

Coping with Chinese torture...Um
I mean mammograms.

Ok ladies, I think we all agree that a man had to have come up with this invention. I had always heard my mother talk about going for her mammogram. She and her little group of buddies made all the regular wisecracks about the joys of getting squished. I was never really afraid to have one, but I knew I was definitely in for an experience when I finally made my way to what I will affectionately call "the machine".

Despite the fear in the air, I struggled to step outside myself and look in on how an event like this must look to the average person. How would I look to someone else while standing there in a modified toga trying to remain modest and dignified with one boob hanging out? Marching up to "the machine" and slapping "it" in there, I began to understand how milk cows might feel. That was the image in my mind anyway. Then it got worse. I never knew my boob could get that flat. I wondered if it would eventually fluff back out. I can also envision a moment when there is a fire alarm and everyone runs out of the office leaving me intimately intertwined with this device. If I wanted to laugh or scream at that moment my hopes were dashed when the technician said, "Don't breathe". I was amazed how good she was at telling me that right after all the air in my lungs had expired. They must have special classes for that.

Oh and I must not forget the toga, or more specifically the lovely modified hospital gowns they provide for you to change into. A departure from the standard hospital gown, these charming fashion statements can be a challenge as they have three armholes. Do you know any women with 3 arms? I certainly don't. I guess they want to be politically correct and provide proper attire for any visiting 3-armed aliens who need mammograms. (If an alien has three arms, how many boobs does it have?) A word to the wise, look for the tag. I managed to get this thing on backwards every time until experience taught me to seek out the tag and make sure it went in the back. If you can't find the tag, well good luck to you. Just put it on, you won't be in it long anyway.

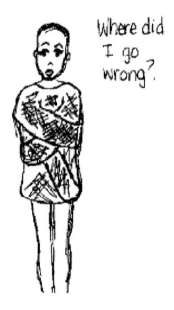

Where did I go wrong?

Did I just get shot?!

If the nurse had not prepared me for the sound of the needle when I had my core biopsy, I certainly would have thought I must have arrived in time for target practice! It is loud, and quite frankly I wondered for a second if a disgruntled ex-employee had wandered into the examining room. A core biopsy is designed to get a significant cross section of tissue by using a hollow needle that removes tissue from the center of the mass. I was still not quite used to people sticking needles in my breast. I would soon learn to get used to it, much to my dismay. I don't think I'd ever get used to this noise. It was a bit of a shock.

They used a sonogram to locate the tumor and then prepared the needle. It sounded like a BB gun and looked a bit like a *Duraflame* lighter. I had very honest medical professionals who explained this procedure fairly thoroughly, and that is invaluable when you have so many questions. My advice to anyone newly diagnosed is to read as much as you can. Arm yourself with knowledge and ask lots of questions so you won't be wondering if someone just nabbed you with a pellet gun.

6

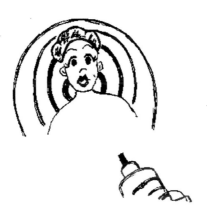

Technology may come and go but hospital gowns remain the same.

Why after all these years, after we send a man to the moon and develop the Internet, why can't they fix those darn hospital gowns? Another word to the wise is prepared for the draft. I know those things provide easy access to key areas, but there has to be a better way. Some kind of panel that snaps, much like those in a pair of long johns would work for me. Not only do we have to be embarrassed for ourselves while wearing these things, we have to be embarrassed for the other patients we inadvertently get to "view". A gal pal of mine in her 50's found herself face to face with the cutest male nurse in the hospital. Cancer and her age did not stop her from flirting incessantly with him until she realized she was completely exposed and hanging out the back of her wheelchair. Suddenly modesty found its way back into her life. What a shame.

Maybe this is really why they give us Morphine in the hospital. It isn't for the pain; it's for the humiliation. Once I was back from surgery and "high on life" I noticed I didn't care so much anymore. I think my family protected me from my temporary lack of modesty. They seemed to keep me covered for visitors and even just for my peace of mind. I suppose they all realized that when I came to my senses I would be mortified to know that my buns had been as much on display as my boob.

A small footnote to this section, my father recently had some outpatient surgery and was instructed to slip into the hospital gown provided. I always knew he was the creative sort and due to the fact that he could not reach around to adequately tie the gown in the back, he solved the dilemma by turning it around and tying it in the front. The hospital staff was quite amused, it seems they had never seen that one done before. Leave it to my family to come up with the unorthodox solution to this dressing dilemma. I'm not sure I recommend this procedure to everyone but it's definitely a thought!

I'm a walking satellite?

If my doctor had not outlined this next procedure in some detail, I would have thought I was in an episode of the "Twilight Zone". They call it wire localization. I call it bizarre. They *did* numb the area and I must admit I barely felt anything through the entire process, but this procedure involved inserting a thin wire into the breast to locate a small questionable mass. Using a sonogram, the wire was then inserted into the mass so that the surgeon would not have to search excessively to locate the area. Sounds reasonable enough, BUT ever sit up with a wire sticking out of your boob? Again I was in no pain, it's just the visual image here that seems a bit extreme. Apparently this is enough to cause women to faint. They kept asking me if I was ok and had a wheelchair standing by.

Just when I thought life couldn't get any weirder. They escort me back to "the machine" for what else? A mammogram. Yes, I have a wire sticking straight out of my breast and they want to stick it in "the machine" and smash it flat again. How did I get to this party? I did look like a human antennae and I did wonder what kind of reception I could get. I could have a whole new career. Some women that have this procedure report being given a Styrofoam cup to cover the end of the wire. I suppose this is to prevent eye injury to the patient or any unsuspecting passersby. I was not given a cup. I think I must have been deprived. It seems they were still waiting for me to faint as people kept asking me if I needed that wheelchair. I proudly proclaimed, "Its my boob not my leg!" and went on to the next adventure.

8

Morphine, breakfast of champions.

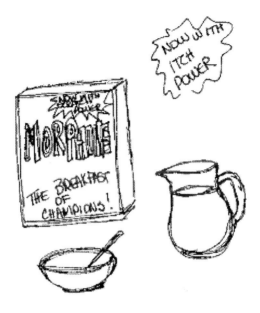

Ahhh, one of the small joys in life, Morphine in the hospital. I remember waking up smiling. I smiled as they rolled me down the hall. I smiled in the elevator. I smiled at complete strangers passing me by. I think I even smiled at the walls. I felt pretty darn good and enjoyed it while it lasted. Of course as with all great things in life, joy turns to nausea pretty quick. For those of us with weak stomachs it happens even quicker. The nurses tried their best to keep my tummy quiet but it would not cooperate. Truthfully I think it best to let the stomach speak its mind and get it all out. Then everyone can get some sleep. (Unless someone staying with you snores.)

One little side note on this wonder drug, you might want to have access to a back scratcher. Actually you may just want a "whole body scratcher". As I began to scratch at the imaginary fleas on my body, a girlfriend of mine explained to me that Morphine makes you itch. It seems to be a side effect of many pain medications. Even my palms itched, and how do you scratch your palms really? Trust me when you try to do that you look a little strange. Want to guess what this girlfriend of mine gave me for Christmas? A back scratcher, what else?

We all knew we'd need support hose someday, but we thought we'd be wearing them on our legs.

Lymphedema (swelling) is a real concern for women who have had axillary dissections in addition to either a lumpectomy or a mastectomy. An axillary dissection involves the removal of lymph nodes under the armpit. Everyone made sure they told me not to overuse my left arm, I mean everyone. Quite honestly I couldn't raise it above chest level for a while, but once I could, being the obstinate person that I am I decided to walk the dog. Brilliant idea, I know. Of course she decided to wrap her leash around my body causing me to shift control to my left arm. She is also a Siberian Husky, and a Husky's job and mission in life is to PULL. So she did. I am not sure if it was that event specifically or combinations of events much like it that caused me to have some mild swelling in my left arm. I had been duly warned to report any swelling to my doctor as soon as possible. Fortunately I at least paid attention to that and let the doctor know quickly.

Though the swelling was extremely mild, my doctor thought it best as a preventative measure to go ahead and get fitted for a compression sleeve. Basically this looks like support hose for your arm. Well it is support hose for your arm, albeit expensive support hose. They say it's made out of a special material and I want to believe that, as much as I paid for it. I must admit though, it felt nice when I put it on. The principle is that the pressure assists the proper drainage of the remaining lymph nodes. Additionally, after surgery there is a "pins and needles" sensation in the back of the arm. Because of its tight fit the sleeve restricts the movement of this tissue and it can feel like quite a relief to keep that "stuff" from moving around. (And that "stuff" was getting flabbier by the day.) I don't wear mine all the time; if I did I would probably get more help moving things around. Next time I have to carry a heavy bag I'll remember that.

Post-Operative care; the stuffed animal phenomenon.

Before and after my surgery I became the proud recipient of an entire menagerie of stuffed animals. I am not sure how to explain this phenomenon; I only know that it exists. People like to give them to you so let them. I found that I actually enjoyed their comfort and sleeping with one in a strategic location under my arm actually provided some pain/pressure relief. I liken this strange occurrence to the same force that propels people to buy you towels or dishes when you get married. It simply is the best choice for the event. No matter how many you have, you can always have more. I tried to rotate them each night so that none of them felt left out. I suppose its frightening to see a grown woman sleeping with a stuffed unicorn or bunny and its even more frightening that she worries about its feelings, but at least I could tell the person who gave it to me that I did indeed have use for it.

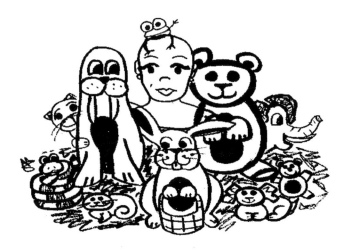

Right before Christmas my husband came home with an early gift for me. He walked in with a giant stuffed Siberian Husky bearing an uncanny resemblance to our "real" dog. This stuffed toy was so realistic that it has on occasion shocked people into wondering what the dog was doing in the house on the bed. This particular Husky doesn't pull anyone's arms out of their sockets either, a big plus! I carried it around for weeks forsaking all other stuffed animals. I know, I know. For shame, for shame! It evened out in the end. Now what I'm going to do with all of these critters I have absolutely no idea. Actually I think I'm going to go get that dog right now. I miss her. How old a woman am I again?

Oh the joy of Christmas...?!

I think everyone felt very concerned that I would have to spend my Christmas holiday recuperating from surgery. On the contrary, if I had to do it, I'm glad that I was able to do so at such a special time of year. It was a joy to look out my hospital window to the oversized lighted Christmas tree below. If you have a choice, I highly recommend scheduling surgery near the holiday. Nurses are less grumpy, doctors are more benevolent and people have time to come and visit you. Lets not forget about holiday fashions either! How many times a year do you get to see nurses sporting smiling Santa's on their frocks? Not to mention receptionists with blinking earrings. Even the doctor's get into the spirit. My surgeon drew a smiling snowman on one of my bandages. It really is the small things that make a difference.

I also racked up in the fleece wardrobe department. Everyone bought me comfort clothes for Christmas. Now I'm a sassy kind of girl myself and usually like to sport more form fitting, sophisticated attire, but at this particular time I was happy for the warm fuzzies I kept getting in all the boxes. Never mind that I did on occasion look like an upright sheep. I was warm and soft, just like the stuffed animal collection I had accumulated. And my husband liked to touch me too, well more like pet me like the dog but who's complaining?

Look out for Jerry Springer! He will suck you in...

Ok, here is the worst problem I faced during my recuperation period. Yes, it was my addiction to Jerry Springer. It wasn't the soap operas I found compelling. I slept during the day. But as I began to channel surf on the television on those sleepless nights, Jerry called to me. I honestly believe that it was the whole concept that I could watch people who have more problems than me. Oh what a terrible thought process, I should be taken out and flogged. Nonetheless I found myself riveted. I was drawn to watch the woman who had to stop her daughter from marrying her former stepfather. I was engulfed in the "Baby, I'm really a man" episodes.

I even began to chant Steve's name when the audience would call for him. But my absolute favorite involved the girl who found her guy cheating with another man while he was wearing a leopard print bra and panties. I know it's not PBS. Some people have drug problems, some people alcohol. I had Jerry Springer.

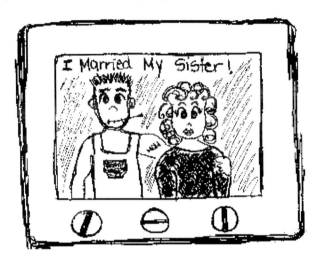

What's worse it that it didn't stop with Jerry Springer. Like a naive person drawn into the world of drugs, I started out on Springer and moved to Court TV. I tried them all; Judge Judy, Curtis Court, Judge Mills Lane. I was addicted to ignorance. I simply had to see whose dog bit whom and which roommate got the boot. I am slowly and gradually weaning myself off of these shows. Nonetheless it is an uphill battle. Once drawn in it is difficult to escape this world. My husband can't understand and I don't expect him to. I am moving in the right direction and soon I will be free of this compulsion. Its like they always say; "...one day at a time."

Chapter Two: Chemotherapy

Have a party...shave your head!

Initially when I began chemotherapy, I cut my hair to prevent the trauma of watching the hair fall out. I believe the hairdresser found it more disturbing than I did; yet it was a bit scary watching the long dark curls fall to the ground. About 10 days into chemo, after doing a daily "testing tug", the hair actually cooperated and came out in small clumps in my hand. A young girl by the name of Asha Mevlana inspired me. I had noticed on her website that she had a head shaving party and shaved the hair before it had a chance to fall out. I decided that was a great way to make the statement that cancer would not get to me, at least not to my spirit. So to the tune of "The Barber of Seville" and "I Think I'm Going Bald" (an obscure Rush song), we shaved the remaining hair off my head. We drank wine and ate pizza and celebrated this "rite of passage" in a defiant way. One little side note, bald may be beautiful, but it is COLD. I never knew how much warmth was retained by that small remaining amount of hair on my head.

I felt free (and chilly), and thankful that I had no big cucumber birthmark on my bald head. Yes I had a nice smooth pate. I realized that I looked pretty good bald, and reveled in that. What a shock after all those years of so much hair. I also discovered that I saved a great deal of money on hairspray and shampoo. But I made up for it in wig expenditures. I also naturally assumed that if I went out bald in public people would know I was on chemotherapy. Wrong! Anyone who had the guts to ask me generally assumed I did this for a fashion statement. What a riot! People thought I would honestly do this to myself on purpose. Still, I would wear my chemo crown with pride when I could and wig wearing became another personal pastime quickly. I changed styles on a whim. Another little gem of wisdom here, buy a good liquid roll on adhesive. Early on I posed the question to my mother that I wondered what I would use to keep my wigs in place. She replied, "Bobby pins, of course!" Think about that for a minute. She still can't believe she said it. The bobby pin has not been made yet that will attach a wig to the bare skull. Think liquid adhesive.

Don't let the cat get your wig!

This is pretty self-explanatory really, however I really had no idea of the appeal of a wig to a cat. I suppose if I really stretch my imagination I can see how it would bear a resemblance to a small rodent. What I wasn't prepared for was coming down the stairs in the middle of the night without my glasses on and finding it lying there waiting for me. Without my very strong spectacles it did appear to be a dead rat. My heart raced and leapt to my throat as I grabbed the banister. Another thing that amazed me is that as I began to relay this story to my friends (thinking it was quite original), I kept getting the comment, "Oh yes! Cat's love wigs." Apparently this is common knowledge, but it was something that my oncologist neglected to mention to me. So I share it with you now. Keep the wigs out of view of the felines. They last longer that way.

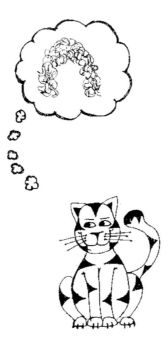

You may want to stay away from the oven while sporting your wig also. Now we all know hair is flammable, and synthetic hair is no exception. But synthetic hair has one quality that human hair does not. Synthetic hair will melt. I heeded my friends' advice as far as using care around candles and the like. I did not however give much thought to the simple process of heating up a pizza. I reached in to the warm oven one night and pulled out my late night snack. I thought no more about it until the next morning when I went to put on my wig. The edges had melted into each other and it was a frazzled mess. Can you say Medusa?

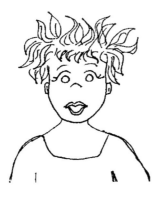

It was virtually unwearable until I ran to a hairdresser to have the edges trimmed off. Apparently it doesn't take much heat to melt a wig. Maybe this would just be a good excuse not to cook until your hair grows out. Let someone else do it while you have a good reason. Take your perks where you can get them.

Make sure they know its YOU!

While we are on the topic of wigs, I must impart to you some additional pearls of wisdom. I have read many books where women are advised to find something very close to their current style and color. Well meaning people will tell you if you are going through chemotherapy to try to make an investment in a high quality wig to minimize the trauma of losing your hair. I say hogwash! How many times have you wanted to try out a new "do" only to chicken out at the last minute or be stopped in your tracks by the fear of change? Here is your excuse to try out every style and color you always wanted. Your bald head is a blank canvas every day. You can pick and choose and not be locked into any one style for too long. Buy inexpensive ones (they look just as good these days) and experiment. You can be blonde on Monday and auburn on Tuesday. I'll admit that the first time I went wig shopping I was a bit overwhelmed. I wish someone had told me this from the start. Rejoice in it! One of the best days I've had of late was when I headed out to the beauty supply store (where you can get lots of cheap wigs) and started trying on hair. In between styles I walked around bald, which led other ladies to come up and talk to me curious about my smooth pate. By the time we were done 4 or 5 of us had tried on every wig in the shop. We laughed constantly and drove the salespeople nuts. Honestly you must try it one day...hair or no hair...its too much fun for a human.

Now I'm lead to mention one other small detail. It is truly liberating to have all of these coiffure choices on a daily basis, but you might want to prepare your friends and family that you have several different looks. Hair is quite an identifying feature and people will not recognize you from time to time. That can also be an advantage, BUT, there are times when it is important for them to know its YOU! One night my husband and I decided to go out for dinner at our favorite restaurant. It is a little family owned Italian eatery, where the owners are apt to sit down with you and chat if the crowd is slow. When we walked in my hubby informed me that he was getting intense stares from the entire staff. He was becoming extremely uncomfortable and it finally dawned on us that they thought he was having an affair with some mysterious exotic blonde. I had to walk up to them and shout, "It's me!" Much laughter and joy ensued. They all said that he would have to be crazy to bring another woman in that place. I know now that I have people to look out for me! So go with it and enjoy your new style, just make sure you tell everyone its you. After all, I wouldn't want anyone to get hurt!

You may be bald but you still have to shave your legs.

Here is one of God's cruel jokes right here. There is no hair on your head or under your arms, your eyebrows are falling out, and you are going bald in unmentionable places, but you STILL have to shave those legs. Now I admit, maybe not quite as often. But this is truly a travesty. What kind of space age polymer is leg hair made of that it resists chemotherapy? Maybe they should consider using this material in road or vehicle construction. No wait! Maybe they can use it to actually make a pair of panty hose that do not run. Wouldn't that be ironic?

They also tell you that you can't afford an infection at this time so you should use a good electric razor. So my family presented one to me for Christmas. I think it might make a good sweater shaver, but I couldn't get it to do much damage on that ever-resistant hair on my legs. I realize I took on the risk of infection to breakdown and use the old aloe strip Bic, and I don't recommend this procedure to you. Razors can be pretty scary when you can't afford a nick or scratch, but I lost my resolve and my sanity when my leg hair began to leave abrasions on my husband's body and it began to shred the sheets. Be careful, use good judgment, and keep the antiseptic nearby.

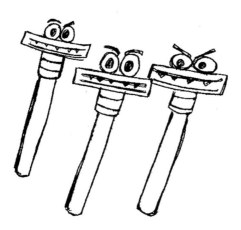

The face is familiar but I can't quite remember my name.

There is something they call "Chemo Brain". It has been studied and it is quite real. Many doctors and professionals are hesitant to talk about it and I don't intend to make light of the challenges it causes. But in all honesty, I've done some pretty ditzy things as of late and I sincerely hope that I can blame it on the "Chemo Brain". Otherwise its senility and I'm not ready for that yet!

You know when you execute a command on a computer and it usually takes a split second to process? When your computer system is running slow or about to crash it just keeps churning and processing. Well my brain began to do that. I'd stare into the refrigerator.... processing, processing. I'd walk into the kitchen...processing, processing. People would ask me what I was doing. "Processing", became my reply. I suppose the best illustration here, and the one my husband will never let me live down, is the night we went shopping at the local superstore. We pulled our cart up to the register, paid for our purchases and my husband gathered all the bags together. We then proceeded to the parking lot with him carrying the bags, and me pushing the *empty* cart straight on to the car. He watched me intently pushing this empty cart out of the store with disbelief. All he said was, "Why?" I had no legitimate answer as I stared blankly back…just processing.

The Legal Way to "Shoot Up"...Drugs Provided!

I never really imagined I'd be the type to shoot myself in the leg with needles. Now I've been a good patient all my life, taking my shots when necessary. But having to jab myself is another story altogether. After my first treatment I was told that I was to be instructed on how to give myself shots. These are designed to make sure blood counts remain high and stable. Chemotherapy does zap your immunity and you become keenly aware of your body's ability to fend off disease. They brought out the little "strap-on" pad designed to look a little like a spot of skin on your leg or arm. I was quite successful at shooting up the little pad; my own leg was an entirely different animal. The faces I made while determining the exact spot to stick myself were akin to those someone might make when constipated.

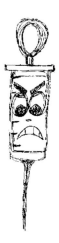

I soon discovered that the shots really did not hurt; it was the imagery that caused me grief. If I found a really nice spot of cellulite I would not even feel it. Unfortunately for me, as is the case most of the time, if there is a side effect I will find it. What I did begin to feel was a rash and swelling as the little "bee sting" shots began to cause a reaction on my legs. The doctor gave me the option to switch to another set of shots that provided the same immune system boost, of course they tend to cause "bone" pain. To itch or to ache that is the question. Well I tried the other shots and a few days later I was happy to go back to itching. At least I could scratch that.

Lose 7 pounds in a day, the chemo way!

Do I really have to elaborate here? Chemotherapy does have its reputation. There are people who say they had mild to non-existent nausea. I was not one of them. I could not keep down water. There are new anti-emetic (nausea) drugs on the market today that are designed to make the process more tolerable. I am sure that they helped me despite my struggle. And believe it or not I was sicker once in my life. Just once, and it involved some very poorly prepared fish. I also had other symptoms that cause you to lose weight at the same time. This will tend to immobilize you. (Get the mental picture? Good!) Some people are able to work through the whole process; I was quite inseparable from my restroom. I actually lost those 7 pounds in one week, although it felt like a day.

I don't mean to frighten anyone; I am just the lucky person who seeks out side effects like a private detective seeks out a cheating spouse. Most doctors will tell you the side effects may include many things. They will rattle out a list that makes the mind reel. Most people don't experience them all and have them to varying degrees. I just had to test them all out so that I could write this book. Side effects of chemo may include: Hair Loss, Dry Mouth, Fatigue, Nausea, Diarrhea, Constipation, Night Sweats, Mouth Ulcers, Hallucinations, Delusions of Grandeur, Anthrax, Smallpox, Bubonic Plague and Leprosy. Oh dear, sorry I got carried away. Would you believe me if I told you its really not that bad? I didn't think so.

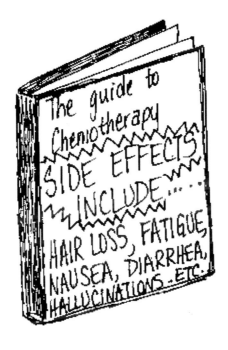

Red Kool Aid may never look the same (ingestible!).

There's a little drug they call Adriamycin. They like to give it to cancer patients. Cancer patients generally don't like it much, though it has this redeeming quality of killing the cancer. It's nice and red just like the Cherry Kool Aid you drank as a kid. Don't let the sweet demeanor fool you. You know the nickname for this stuff, hmmm? Yes they call it the "Red Devil". This stuff can make you toss your cookies faster than you can say blech. Many folks swear to this day they can't even look at Cherry Kool Aid. I of course professed to the nurse that I could delineate between a drug to treat me for cancer and a sweet refreshing summertime treat. What bravado. Guess what? I can't even look at the stuff without wanting Compazine (for nausea). And I'm allergic to Compazine.

While I'm on the topic of such craziness, I was surprised to learn that the first chemotherapy drugs were derived from Mustard Gas. Amazing that there really seems to be two sides to every coin. Chemical warfare, designed to immobilize, actually has the inherent quality of killing cancer cells. What an eye opening concept and one that causes pause for thought. Well not such a completely novel thought. Penicillin came from mold. I wonder what kind of heinous disease I could cure from not cleaning out my refrigerator. Maybe I'll stop doing it in the name of science.

If at all possible buy stock in Ginger Ale.

Ginger Ale probably saved my life as much as anything else did. Clear and bubbly, it soothes the savage tummy. If I could have been hooked to an IV of it I probably would have done so. I know it's the ginger in it that does the trick, but that carbonation helps. My mother and I got smart and thought we would try ginger tea also. Well sometimes hot liquids in bed are not the smartest idea. I sported a small burn on my leg for a while from that little disaster. I suppose it helped my stomach, but my leg hurt so bad I didn't think of much else for a while. If you want to try the tea just use the kitchen table.

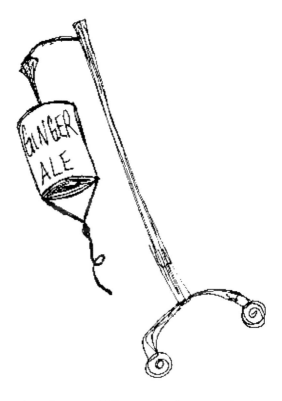

Like fine wines there are differences in the taste of various ginger ale's. You may wish to sample different ones to find the taste that suits you best. Some are drier, some are bubblier. I found that I preferred the cans to bottles. That was just a matter of personal taste. I became a veritable connoisseur of ginger ale. I found that for nausea related matters it was best served at room temperature and fresh. However, this bubbly ale does have a longer shelf life than its darker cola counterparts and is perfect for leaving by the beside for late night medications. Just be advised you might go beyond the dainty burping that ladies generally manage. My husband swears he's duct taped all the pictures to the walls to prevent me from shattering them.

The Portal Catheter, your third nipple. Learn to love it.

I know that's a lovely mental image but there is no getting around it. My "port" as they call it is a Godsend. Implanted just beneath the surface of my skin near my breast, it serves as the location for blood work and IV administration. How much easier it is that having someone poke at my arm? It is virtually painless too. I highly recommend them but they make dressing a challenge. No more spaghetti strapped dresses and plunging necklines for a while. I have had quite the love/hate relationship with this little devil.

Other points you may wish to be aware of? Its metal, which gets cold in the winter, very cold. Scarves are an excellent addition to the wardrobe because of this. It was a little itchy in the summer. Also, since it is metal I have the dubious distinction of being able to set off a metal detector. It is almost as charming as having a metal plate in my head. Actually I guess it could make for interesting conversation. "You have a metal what?" After its removal I'm planning on having a little butterfly tattoo placed over the small scar as a symbolic reminder of what was once there.

Chapter Three: Radiation

A new concept in tanning.

I was so thankful that I had a reprieve from chemo that I looked at radiation as a vacation. And so it was for a while, complete with tanning apparatus. Unfortunately it wasn't a full body tan, no, just a little exercise in "spot tanning". And never before did I have "tanning therapists" present when I went to radiate myself. Usually it was just a little more private than this, but that's ok, they seemed to know what they were doing.

Still I missed the hum of the tanning bed as opposed to the whir of the radiation equipment. I also missed a bit of the privacy. If I wanted to tan "au naturel" before it was just that bed and I. Now I had people hovering. What cracks me up is that of course I had to don the gown with 3 armholes to get into the room, but they left one side of me covered up. Excuse me but if you are thoroughly examining my left breast do you think the right one is that much worse? If for some reason the gown slipped off of the adjoining breast they quickly covered it back up. What strange logic is there in this? You know I'm a package deal; they pretty much go together, my breasts. I kept thinking one day I was going to rip off the gown completely and shout, "Made you look!". I'm glad I didn't. I might have wound up in a padded room."

I don't bend that way!

You know how you used to bend your Barbie doll in positions that no human being could possibly get into? Then when you tried it yourself you wound up in the emergency room? Well no one told the therapists who measured me and fit me with my radiation mould about this. It would have been nice if they had done so. I wound up in a contorted state for an hour praying for Tylenol (with codeine). Ok, ok it wasn't that bad. It's just that us gals who just had axillary dissections don't really like to raise our arms above our heads, and that is exactly what they made me do. I kept telling myself that cramps had to be worse than laying with my arm over my head, but I wasn't very good at convincing myself.

Here's another bizarre experience. When you get measured for radiation they take a big garbage bag and fill it with cement and make you lay in it. Ok not really, but it looks like a garbage bag and they do put goo in it. Then you have to be still, very still. The mould hardens around you and this way they are very exact in treating the same location every time. So you lay there half naked in goo, perfectly still, in moderate pain, thinking this is interesting.

Tic-Tac-Toe anyone?

Then they take a big permanent magic marker and draw on you. Honestly this felt like some crazy kindergarten craft experiment gone awry. (Remember when you used to lay down and the teacher would trace your body on paper? We cut them out and carried them around?) So they drew and drew and drew. It felt a little odd, in fact it tickled. I couldn't see this incredible work they were creating though, which made the experience even more unnerving. Some women are given small tattoos to help guide the therapists. Either way our bodies are true works of modern art. My radiation oncologist came into the room to check on the progress. He said, much to my disbelief, "You look beautiful!" What a comedian. I retorted back, "I can only imagine!" They finally finished with me, the "human graph paper", and let me go get dressed.

When I looked in the mirror, there were lines from my neck, extending to my upper arm and down my belly. I was a human tic-tac toe board. Thank God they took the lines off my neck before I walked out. I could just hear people stopping me in the grocery store saying; "I'll take the center square to block!" I couldn't wait to go home and show my husband my kinky new look. He took one look and said with his rapier sharp wit that he thought I was two letters away from hangman. I began to think maybe I could get a job as a human bingo card. There is nothing else I can say; it really was an experience too weird for words.

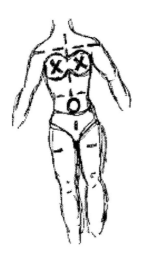

Remain seated until the ride has come to a complete stop.

If I was thinking it, the therapist said it. The "table" that they place you on to treat you is a marvel of modern science. It slides back and rises up much like a ride at your favorite amusement park. So when the therapist said, "Please keep your hands and arms inside until the ride has come to a complete stop." I had already been there in my mind. That was the most fun part of my daily treatments. I looked forward to my brief ride everyday. They belted me in too, just like the staff at Disney World.

Of course once the ride reaches the top, they leave you sitting there like they do on the Ferris wheel. You are stuck and belted in. Might as well enjoy the ride. I made the comment once that I might just go to sleep while they fussed around me. I was told they would charge rent if I slept. You get no sympathy sometimes. Speaking of fussing, boy do they flit around you, pushing in this thing and pulling out that one. Snapping things in and turning them around. I'm not sure if they were really working or just doing stuff that looked complicated to impress me. It worked; I couldn't remember all that with my chemo brain. I'd be radiating the fibers in the carpet before I could get it right.

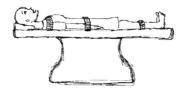

The laser light show!

As if to continue to try to impress me with the dramatic effect of it all, they turn off the lights. It's like going to the planetarium. They line up lasers along the areas to be treated. If you look up to the ceiling you see a bright red eyeball looking down at you. Yes I know it's a laser, but it reminds me of some Stephen King novel my husband likes to read. It just sits there watching you like big brother. Maybe they put it there to intimidate you into laying still. The big red eyeball knows all. I would try to ignore it but its like the Mona Lisa, anywhere you move your eyes you can still feel it looking at you, following you. It's a little spooky.

Then they leave me all alone in the room with the eyeball. As they leave they pass through a curtain that they slide quickly shut. This has an eerie "Wizard of Oz" effect. Should I really pay no attention to the man behind the curtain? He sure is making a lot of odd noises in there. He could be planning to launch me into outer space as the machine fires up and I hear its engine roar. Perhaps I have an overactive imagination? Still what the heck do they do back there? The world may never know.

Who ya gonna call?

The table may bear a resemblance to a fun park ride, whereas the entire apparatus bears a striking resemblance to a giant telephone. Yes it's a room-sized telephone and the top part of the handset rotates. I get the feeling you could call Guam without much difficulty with a phone this size. Maybe its there so you can have a direct line to the "Big Guy". I could call up God and say, "Hey can we talk about this cancer thing?" I bet the long distance bill would be huge though. (Oh I know it's a bad joke, humor me!)

The first day I saw it actually the system was down for maintenance. I could see all the "spaghetti" in between the pieces of equipment. For a moment I heard an operator's voice in the back of my head that said, "We're sorry, your call did not go through, please try your call again later." I wanted to ask if the telephone repairman was in the building, but you know I doubt they would have appreciated that too much.

Where is the Solarcaine?

I wasn't feeling a thing there for a while, just getting in and out as quickly as possible. Then I started getting my sunburn. I looked like the Coppertone girl, only a little more extreme and in reverse. I doubt that winds up on a billboard anytime soon! I was suddenly thankful I had gone to the tanning bed in the buff over the last couple of years, as I hoped that it would toughen up that skin that never sees the light of day. Still I'm a fair skinned gal, I knew I was in for some "fun in the sun" before this was over.

They gave me several creams to use and I tried to use them liberally at home. They were moderately effective. But for some reason this year in April the weather decided to go haywire. It got to 90 degrees before the middle of the month. This did not help my dressing dilemma. I couldn't expose the treated shoulder to the sun, but the heat made anything I wore over the area unbearable. I had found myself in a true Catch-22 situation. So...I took to walking topless around the house. My husband found this fascinating, but I had to use extreme caution around the bay window in the kitchen and the front door. I doubt my neighbors would understand my "flashy" behavior. Again avoiding the oven in this state is also probably wise. Be lazy, order takeout.

Is that gum in your mouth?

I have heard from patients that have been reprimanded for chewing gum in the radiation room. They want you to be perfectly still, no gum chewing allowed. One lady even suggested that she was afraid to keep the gum in her mouth after she realized she had been chewing it in the event that it had picked up extra gamma rays and started glowing in the dark recesses of her mouth. It is interesting the ideas that we all have about radiation and its "dangerous effects". Many of us watch the therapists scurry out of the room like mice right before they zap us. And they tell us this is going to make us healthy again? Why do they run like that?

I was quite proud of my ability to keep very still. I think I learned it while doing freeze modeling many years ago. While modeling swimwear in a department store I was able to stay very stiff and not even blink. Unfortunately that caused my eyes to dry out and one of my contact lenses fell out on the other model's arm. It was very embarrassing. But I drew on that experience in radiation. The therapists marveled at the day when a stack of moulds fell off the wall shelf onto the floor causing a loud clash. I never flinched. Not even 5 minutes later I had to sneeze while a treatment was being administered. I barely blinked my eyes. When finished I walked out to the praise and adoration of my caregivers. It was a proud moment. I think it also helps that I have animals in the house and am quite used to hearing loud crashes at any given time during the day. Draw on the skills you know you have.

They drew on me again!

Just when I thought those lines were fading for good they had to "re-measure" me for my final treatments. Many times they will give patients a "boost" very specific to the area where the cancer was located. So they drew a big oblong circle on me this time, and golly doing it once just wasn't enough. One therapist/artist drew around it again, fearing the first marker might not be as permanent. Oh my! Did it ever tickle? It made me wonder if this was how Goldie Hawn must have felt when they drew all over her for those old "Laugh In" episodes. (She did giggle a lot.) At any rate when I went home to show my husband the artwork this time his quip was even better. He threatened to write in the circle "Place hands here", as if this is some bizarre body map. Honestly, this is what I had to put up with.

At this point my burns had begun healing in areas that had stopped receiving radiation. Still I sported a strange shaped tan on my back. My chest did not burn as much as my shoulder and back. It seems the "exit" site, or site where the radiation leaves the body gets burned in frequent cases. Of course this had to be the year of halter-tops and sundresses and I had the challenge of dressing around the trapezoidal tan on my back. One man who decided to point this out to me (because of course I couldn't possibly know) wanted to know why I had these markings. I just told him that aliens were zapping me with their ray guns. That shut him up pretty quick.

Applause, Applause!

Being a theatre buff, vocalist and diva (my friends have bestowed me this title), I live for applause. So maybe even better than getting applause from a performance is getting applause for laying on a table for 6 weeks. I must admit I was happy to finish that daily trek to the doctor's office, though I truly loved the staff. They clapped for me and we all shouted for joy when the last whir was done. One wise guy even offered me my mould. I'm sure you can imagine what I told him he could do with it.

Chapter Four: Chemo the Sequel

Just When you Thought it was Safe

It was the great wisdom of my doctors that called for me to take additional chemotherapy treatments. They use this sandwich technique to make sure that you are not delayed too long in receiving one treatment as opposed to another. I can't say I was jumping for joy at the prospect of more chemotherapy, but I would take any other weapon they would give me in my arsenal to fight cancer. This time the magic potion was Taxol.

That being said, I marched back up to the Oncologist's office to "take my medicine". This time going into the office I felt very comfortable, almost home away from home. I had worked with my oncologist and my radiation oncologist on the *Relay for Life* during my little reprieve from radiation. I guess you could say worked. It seems I helped chair the luncheon and the survivors' tent at the relay, walked the first lap, jumped up and sang a set, got hugged by Tammy Faye, danced the Macarena and the Electric Slide, played another set, and played DJ after the DJ left. (Oh I did run home for one errand at which time my cat got out and I had to chase her for twenty minutes around the yard at 6am). I was completely tuckered! Needless to say I also got to know all the medical professionals I've been seeing for months now even better. They probably got to know me more intensely than they cared to. So on that first day back for chemo my family and I annoyed everyone in the chemo room with pictures of the event, videos of newscasts and stories of the docs and the relay. It's a good thing we had all that stuff, this transfusion took forever. But the Benadryl was nice, it probably saved us all by keeping me mellow.

Hey I didn't toss my cookies?

What, you say, no nausea? Ok well a little nausea, but no worshipping the god of porcelain on this go round. I was almost disappointed. I thought I might lose 5 pounds. Well, I wasn't really disappointed but I was shocked. They did tell me that Taxol was much easier than Adriamycin and it turns out to be true, at least for me. So even though I didn't have much taste I relished the fact that I could in fact take a little pleasure in food. And did I mention no shots? Oh it was a great day when I realized I wouldn't have to poke myself daily for the sake of my blood counts.

36

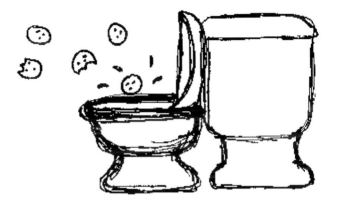

Oh yes and weeks into treatment there was something else I wasn't counting on, HAIR. It was still growing. Every day I pulled it and every day it hurt. And that made me happy. (Yes I'm a sick puppy I know.) As long as it hurt I knew it wasn't falling out. Now let me clarify, I still had my wig fetish and rightfully so. Yes I had hair but I looked like Drew Carey. I even have the horned rimmed reading glasses to complete the effect. This look didn't really work for me so I stuck with the wigs; they were a little more alluring. The only thing I'd like to have of Drew's is his money, certainly not his fashion sense. (No offense Drew.)

I've Fallen and I Can't Get Up!

The one side effect that I did begin to notice was a little joint and muscle pain. I had been sent to the GNC store by my doctor to buy Glutamine from the very muscular woman who I am quite sure could have pummeled me into the ground with her pinky. I do believe the Glutamine prevented some pain, I hope so because it cost more than several doctor's visits combined. I also wouldn't want to make "Greta the Glutamine Goddess" angry by saying her product didn't work. Still I did feel a little achy, like I had the flu.

A friend of ours called and invited us to their pool. I thought that would be a great way to soothe my muscles.

Off we went to frolic in the wonderful land of above ground pools. I was having such a great time seeing friends, having a little wine, when suddenly as if decreed by the gods, one of the boards on the deck suddenly collapsed under the intense pressure of my 133 pounds. (Yes that is sarcasm there.) The ground just opened up and swallowed my left leg. I had indeed fallen and I was having some degree of difficulty getting up. All the fellows at the party insisted I just wanted their attention. I insist that the board ate my leg and did not want to give it back. And oh you should have seen it, there it was bruised and scraped in a heinous manner. I looked like I'd had some bizarre abstract tattoo work done on my entire leg. Good thing I had that wine, I'm sure it helped me not be too concerned for the pain, at least not until the next day. And wouldn't my oncologist just kill me…

I guess I should mention…

Up until this point I have neglected to mention that in my infinite wisdom I decided to enter a beauty pageant while undergoing all this treatment. Not the choice of the typical chemo patient mind you, but the Global America pageant was a fund raiser for Breast Cancer so I felt like it was a great way to raise awareness, by competing while on treatment. I'd show the world that we are all still vital and powerful. Still shopping for outfits to match the right wig (and now to cover up my disfigured leg) was getting to be tedious. I coated myself nightly with self-tanner so I didn't reflect the standard chemo pallor. God forbid I should get in front of those lights and be so white people would need sunglasses to see me. Oh and the hair I mentioned earlier, forget it! It started coming out again. So preparing for the pageant meant another good shave too. A word of advice, no matter how desperate you are to get that hair out of your head, stay away from the Lady Bic. That isn't what they were meant for. What a mess I made. I looked like I was wearing a hair beanie. One good thing about remaining stubble however is that it makes great Velcro for holding on a wig. I didn't use the liquid adhesive once and I took home 1st runner up, talent and get this… photogenic. Yes, photogenic, using none other than my bald picture. So don't ever tell me that bald isn't beautiful.

From Crowning to Chemo.

I really didn't want to come home from having all that fun to come right back to the oncologist office for chemo, but best to get it out of the way. After this one, I would only have two more. I realized as I sat there this time, looking around, how much this had become home away from home. I took over the room, took my shoes off, got things instead of asking for them. (Sometimes reminded the nurses I needed certain things). I was by all accounts obnoxious. Other patients probably prayed privately that we would shut up so they could get some sleep. I did take in my crown and sashes and plaques from the pageant. I had to show them to someone.

Most of all I had gotten quite adept at unplugging my IV so that I might roll it down to the restroom with me. They pump all that fluid through you and how anyone sleeps I'll never know. My bladder just keeps churning away, making sure I never rest. Back and forth I would scuttle with this thing, wishing we weren't chained together as we were. One doctor in seeing me bustling down the hall said to me, "Only two more times back here with your dance partner huh?" I realized that this thing did bear a resemblance to a hat rack once used by Fred Astaire. "Yes", I replied, "but at least I get to lead!"

Wig Stands?

My mother picks on me incessantly about my choices for places to rest my wigs. Of course the first place I started leaving them instigated the title for this book. I learned not to leave them at the head of the banister. But, lampshades make excellent wig stands. Just don't turn the light on high beam and forget the wig is there. (I did mention the melt factor.) I have a hat stand covered in wigs and it works well. There is a Madonna statuette on my dresser I'm ashamed to admit has held them from time to time. Bedposts are excellent but awfully accessible to the aforementioned felines. My most convenient and creative location as of late however, had to be when I just got fed up at chemo and took the thing off and hung it on my IV. It was perfect. More than one patient got a chuckle as I tripped giddily by them on my way to the bathroom, bald, rolling my IV with the wig decorating the top. Just take a moment and visualize if you can.

Strike That, Reverse It...

Well I had become accustomed to that bizarre logic that said "you shall have no hair on your head but you must shave your legs." I think the general idea here was to constantly confuse the patient on as regular a basis as possible. I may not have hung on to that new hair that had been sprouting, still little tufts kept trying to shoot up at any rate. But now as I got ready to rid my body of all other unwanted hair I found that there was my surprise, NO HAIR ON MY LEGS. This was quite the reverse of my expectations. Smooth as a baby's bum, I didn't have to shave for months. I found myself from time to time even running my hands across the stubble free skin. I figured it would be a long time before I would ever have that experience again. As much as I enjoyed it I still don't plan on ever ordering that stuff of the television that wipes off hair with a washcloth. No when my hair comes back I'll be content to shave it. Just one more way of instigating my return to a "semi-normal" life. Have razor, will shave.

We All Look Alike.

Having been bald for going on eight months I found that I racked up all kinds of comments from friends and strangers. Some of them fairly original but sadly many of them repeated themselves. Demi Moore was never actually bald but I guess she must have had a good shaped head so people would tell me I looked just like her. (Right, that's why I have all those agents beating down my door.) Sinead O'Connor was of course another obvious comparison. Being a vocalist everyone quipped that I should add "Nothing Compares 2 U" to my repertoire. But the most common comparison I seemed to get was...drum roll please..."You look just like that chick from Star Trek". Yes it seems that there has been one identifiable attractive bald chick in our country's culture. Since she is the only one most people remember, all attractive bald chicks who follow will undoubtedly be compared to her. I would make some silly comment about getting the "carbon based life forms" out of my way and smile. How could I be upset, the girl was gorgeous. It may be the last time in my life someone compares me to such a model. So I'll take the compliment I suppose. Now if you'll excuse me I think "V'ger" is calling me.

Top Ten?

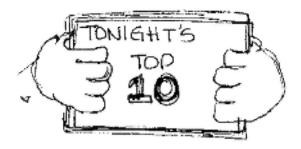

At this point we've tried to examine the good side to all this insanity. I thought this might be a good time to officially list some of the finer points of chemotherapy treatment. Am I sick and twisted? Definitely.

Top Ten Advantages of Chemotherapy Treatment:

10. You save money on Slim Fast.
9. No need to hide from your enemies, they won't recognize you.
8. Shampoo? What's that?
7. Razor burn? What's that?
6. Ticks are easy to spot on your head.
5. Super anti-nausea drugs are great for a hangover.
4. Hare Krishnas don't approach you at the airport.
3. You don't have to clean your hairbrush.
2. Even mosquitoes don't want your blood.
1. NO bad hair days.

That's it? Now What?

The day finally arrived when I was to have my last chemotherapy treatment, but due to some nerve damage in my hands and feet from this medication, they decided to cancel the last treatment. So my last chemo appointment was a brief physical exam and private conversation with my doctor. (Who said I was one of his favorites because he never knew who I was going to be when he saw me.) After all of this craziness I was done, finished, through. Whenever I have finished with a performance for most of my life, applause usually follows. I was so ecstatic to be through that I happily paid the receptionist and told the nurses I would see them in six weeks for a check up. Then I went home. No applause, no confetti, no party…it was just quiet. What a shock, is this what I worked for? Now what do I do?

I realized at that moment that it was up to me to celebrate for myself the milestone that I had just reached. No one else, no matter how close to you they are can know what it means to you. The next day, my oncologist sent me balloons and cookies. And I appreciated them all the more because of that self realization. (And the cookies had chocolate in them!) I also realized I had to take baby steps to resume certain roles in my own life. I felt like everyone looked at me saying "Ok, now you are done, get back to work." It takes more time than that to heal, allow yourself that. Besides I get to take Tamoxifen now and menopause will be my next adventure! Well maybe we should call it "Tamoxipause"? Lucky me, I'll more than likely get to experience menopause twice. If something is worth doing, I suppose its worth doing again? Hey at least I won't miss the cramps.

Chapter Five: Random Moments of Joy

Let Me Explain…

I wanted to make sure when I wrote this book that other women had experienced similar experiences with "hair humor" and the like. It turns out that I was not alone. I belong to a forum for Breast Cancer survivors online.   When I asked for humorous anecdotes to share in my book, I was regaled with some of the most amusing stories I have ever heard. Included here are some of the best. The names have been withheld to protect the innocent.

Pirates!

[One] weekend, "Jim" and I were grocery shopping.. We both had bandannas on, both black and white. We were coming out of the store and this lady and her young son were walking in front of us. He was about 3 1/2 yrs old. As they were walking he turned around and looked at "Jim" and I. His eyes got really big. The little boy then said to his mom, "Mommy, Mommy look! There are pirates in this store." Well, "Jim" and I thought this was so cute. His mom did the mom thing, "Yes, yes, ok, ok", but did not even turn around. He kept saying, "Mommy, look pirates!", she never did turn around and this poor kid thought pirates were following him.

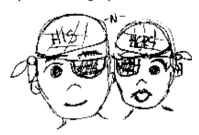

Rock'em Sock'em!

Would you like to hear about my first prosthesis? Before I could get to a town big enough to carry such things I made do with not just a sock, as some have. I wanted weight too, so I used a good sized rock. One I had collected from somewhere...a nice big agate. I wore my "rock-sock" boob and warned everyone who gave me a hug!

Mexican Surprise?

Having all my "work" done in Mexico and not speaking Spanish was a challenge. Like the time I was in for my diagnostic testing...the sweet man doing my liver scan motioned me to push up my shirt, so I did. I raised it all the way to my neck exposing both 50 yr. old-seen-better-days boobs. He quickly pulled my shirt back down to my midriff. "Oops", says I, "so sorry to show more than needed". I was just in phase "one" then and not at all used to "showing off".

The Price is Right...

When my hair started growing after chemo, I bought one of those little clip-on ponytails to make it look longer. I just wanted so desperately to look like myself again. I went to Best Buy for CD's and the guys were all looking at me. I felt great (this cancer didn't hurt my looks any, right?). Well finally one of them approached me and told me I had a big yellow price tag (49.95) still on it. I removed the price tag and put the hairpiece back on in my car. Then we saw a guy my husband and I know and I was laughing at one of his stories when the d*** thing fell off and was lying on the floor like some dead rat with a black ribbon around it. I just picked it up off the floor, stuffed it in my handbag and yelled, "See 'ya later", then ran red-faced to my car.

Weight of the World...

A friend was working in her garden. Along side her was her 5 year old daughter. As she bent down to pull a weed, her prosthesis fell out,"plop", in the garden. The daughter picked it up and said, "Hey Mum your shoulder pad has fallen out. Gee, Dad is right, you *have* got the world's weight on your shoulders."

Hair Today?

When I was getting fitted for my wig my hair started falling out. The wig had these little combs in the front to hold it on and when it came off it took a big wad of hair with it. That was a big surprise. (I always thought wigs were supposed to add hair, not take it away!)

Waiter, There's a What in my Soup?

Shortly after surgery the kids visited and wanted to take us out for dinner. My surgery was giving me lots of trouble so I had not gone to be fitted for proper garments. Being a seamstress for years I decided I could solve this problem and make my own makeshift bra. I went to work at sewing this soft padded boob for my first trip into public. I was so proud of myself that I had solved another hurdle in this fight for survival to look normal. I put it into my sports bra and bingo.... worked perfectly.

We were sitting at the table ordering our food when I noticed our new son in law sitting across from me moving his eyes trying to tell me something. I didn't understand. Finally he whispered across the table "Mom you are a little unbalanced." I was crushed and I could see he was uncomfortable. How could he say something like that? I was in complete control of my faculties! Cancer hadn't changed my brain. He watched me for a minute or two and then finally said, "Mom catch your cleavage before it falls in your soup!" I looked down. Oh my gosh there was my boob sitting on the top of my scoop collar. I was so numb from surgery I had not felt it work its way up. After that I learned the skill of securing and weighting my boob.

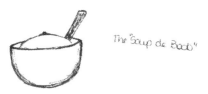

The "Soup de Boob"

Bend-o-Boob...

I decided to just go to the Cancer Center here and "borrow" a prostheses after my mastectomy, because I thought I was going to have reconstruction done in a few months. I am in there and this girl is trying to fit me with a "boob". Finally she finds one "big" enough, and away I go! Well it was a very old prostheses, and it started to bend in half. I looked down one day in the grocery store, and "oops", while one boob was in place the other boob had bent in half! I wondered why people were looking at me funny. Needless to say I went and "purchased" a new one the very next day!

46

Fly and be free?

My oncologist never gives me a gown, she just un-hooks my bra, checks me then hooks me back up. One day as I was leaving there I felt my bra "unsnap". I thought no big deal until the strap slid off my shoulder, my prosthesis ended up on my tummy. I had to walk through a lobby full of people with one boob on my tummy and one on my chest. Bet that blew them away !

Fundies!

While I was going through chemo, I came down with a nasty virus my body couldn't fight. I was running a 104-degree temperature so the Dr. told my family to transport me via an ambulance to the hospital. Since in the heat of my fever I had thrown off most of my clothes, my hubby told my oldest daughter to get some clothes on me before the ambulance got here. She brought some undies in to me and told me to put them on and she would be back with clean pajamas. Well when she came back to room, I had my panties on my head with my ears sticking out the leg holes. I must of thought it was one of my hats to keep my bald head covered. She laughed so hard the rest of the family came to see what was wrong. I don't remember a thing. They felt bad laughing cause I was so sick, but said I really looked funny. Thank goodness they didn't take any blackmail pics.

Soap on a Dope!

When my mother-in-law had her mastectomy she opted for prosthesis over reconstruction. Each night after coming home from work she would pop it out and throw it into the bathtub to await its morning shower. One morning my 80-year-old father-in-law got into the shower first. For 15 minutes my mother-in-law heard mumbling and cussing coming from the bathroom. When my father-in-law emerged, his first words to my mother-in-law were "Ethel, never, ever, ever buy that soap in the bathtub again. It doesn't lather for s***!"

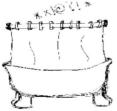

About the Author:

Lauren Brower is a Breast Cancer Survivor living in Charlotte, NC. She was diagnosed at age 34 when her husband discovered a lump on their anniversary. After undergoing surgery, chemotherapy and radiation, her cancer is assumed to be currently in remission.

She was the 2001 Mrs. Central NC representative for the Global America Pageant a pageant that supports breast cancer awareness. Brower was the first contestant to compete while continuing her chemotherapy treatments. She is also involved in a group called the "Young Survivors Coalition", a non-profit organization that focuses on the unique issues and challenges faced by women 40 and under diagnosed with breast cancer.

Mrs. Brower is a professional vocalist and works within the Charlotte community to entertain and enlighten others with her experience.

To contact the YSC: Box 528, 52A Carmine Street
New York, New York 10014
www.youngsurvival.org